# Auras, Chakras, and Energy Fields

# Auras, Chakras, and Energy Fields

✦

## What They Are To You and How Your Angels and Guides Work Through Them

*Sylvia Lavey*

iUniverse, Inc.
New York  Lincoln  Shanghai

# Auras, Chakras, and Energy Fields
## What They Are To You and How Your Angels and Guides Work Through Them

Copyright © 2007 by Sylvia Lavey

All rights reserved. No part of this book may be used or reproduced by any means, graphic, electronic, or mechanical, including photocopying, recording, taping or by any information storage retrieval system without the written permission of the publisher except in the case of brief quotations embodied in critical articles and reviews.

iUniverse books may be ordered through booksellers or by contacting:

iUniverse
2021 Pine Lake Road, Suite 100
Lincoln, NE 68512
www.iuniverse.com
1-800-Authors (1-800-288-4677)

Because of the dynamic nature of the Internet, any Web addresses or links contained in this book may have changed since publication and may no longer be valid.

The views expressed in this work are solely those of the author and do not necessarily reflect the views of the publisher, and the publisher hereby disclaims any responsibility for them.

ISBN: 978-0-595-43627-9 (pbk)
ISBN: 978-0-595-87952-6 (ebk)

Printed in the United States of America

# *Contents*

| | | |
|---|---|---|
| Note | | vii |
| Chapter 1 | Auras and Chakras—What They Look Like | 3 |
| Chapter 2 | Aura Experiences | 11 |
| Chapter 3 | Seeing and Feeling Auras | 17 |
| Chapter 4 | A Healthy Aura Means a Healthy Body | 25 |
| Chapter 5 | Energy Patterns | 29 |
| Chapter 6 | Cause and Affect: Thoughts Create Actions | 41 |
| Chapter 7 | Dreams, Past Lives, or Night Travels? | 53 |
| Chapter 8 | Magic in the Air | 63 |

# *Note*

Human beings have always marveled at their conquests in being able to conquer one continent after another, or travel and explore celestial planets, but few give little thought as to what lies within their very being their soul and their spirit.

For these two areas are where the real conquests exist, and where each person can find the real meaning to life, not as we have been told by society, but what we know through experience from what is, and what has been, that will make the real difference within ourselves and in the long run within every society on this planet and beyond.

Until each human being can fully understand themselves by knowing what lies within, there can be no real peace within or without.

It is through peace that the divine dwells, where real assistance takes place, and where miracles happen.

Sylvia Lavey
Author

*"We are what we repeatedly do."*

—Aristotle (384 BC–322 BC)
Ancient Greek Philosopher, Scientist and Physician

# 1

## *Auras and Chakras—What They Look Like*

Everything around us is made-up of energy. In chapter three of my book titled *Synchronicity* I mention how philosophy views this very concept.

In fact, the human body could be thought of as being electrical energy. Impulses that carry signals throughout the human body carry messages that help govern the life inside and outside of our bodies.

The physical body also has a subtle body (or ethereal body), an aura, and it extends out two or more feet from the physical body in most healthy people. Not everyone can see it so they are not aware of its existence. But, most people have felt it, especially when someone gets too close and their energy is not compatible. This is usually because the other person is ill, uses drugs, over indulges in alcohol, or from karma. Human instinct is to move away immediately, out of the other person's energy field when this happens.

It is the subtle body that makes up the human aura that is fed through the chakras. It envelops the physical body through various layers. Much like the layers of our physical body which has a skeleton, soft tissue, and skin, the ethereal body has it own layers and each layer is a different color. Every person's ethereal body is different, just as no two people have the same physical make-up.

There are seven, well known, major chakras that are part of the human body. They project out two or more feet to help form the human aura. Following is a brief description:

1. Crown chakra on the top of the head–its color is usually white, but most often is seen as violet–it projects straight up into the air and down through the spine. (Known as the Seventh chakra in the human body).

2. Brow chakra in the middle of the forehead–its color is mostly indigo–it projects forward as well as backward through the head. (Known as the Sixth chakra in the human body).

3. Throat chakra in the middle of the throat–its color is mostly medium to light blue–it projects forward and backward through the neck. (Known as the Fifth chakra in the human body).

4. Heart chakra in the chest area–its color is mostly a medium green–it projects forward and backward through the torso. (Known as the Fourth chakra in the human body).

5. Stomach/solar plexus area–its color is mostly yellow–it projects forward and backward through the torso. (Known as the Third chakra in the human body).

6. Abdomen/navel area chakra–its color is mostly orange–it projects forward and backward through the body. (Known as the Second chakra in the human body).

7. End of the spine /root chakra–its color can be mostly red or black–it projects down through the body. (Known as the First chakra in the human body).

The chakras in the human body are known by their numbers according to how close they are from the surface of the earth.

The earth's gravity keeps the human body grounded, which forms a relationship between the human body and the earth.

The colors of the chakras and the aura have a luminous shiny color to them, since the energy they are made up from is ethereal matter.

The seven *major* chakras appear similar to an open flower in the body, but their energy is projected out from the physical body through vortexes into the aura. The energies from the chakras actually look similar to that of small tornados with the very tip being attached to the body, and the open funnel part twisting outward. Since the chakras are constantly moving, spinning, their flower-like shape within the body can be likened to that of a wheel.

So, is it any wonder that when you are around certain people you feel drained; especially if they are ill or are suckers (some people actually feed off other people's energies)?

The body's aura is made up from *major* chakra energies and other energies from *minor* chakras. The *minor* chakras are scattered throughout the torso and head, and are located in the knees, palms of the hands and the arches of the feet.

I first became aware of the chakras in my body in the mid 1970's when I started taking yoga classes. Through meditation and breathing techniques I was able to feel them. This *did not* happen while I was in any of my classes, but while I was meditating alone at home.

In addition, having heard lectures on chakras and the human aura, as well as the experiences mentioned in my book *Synchronicity,* all helped make me more aware of the energy fields around me, and I began to actually see my chakras and their colors.

I remember while meditating one time and thinking that I wanted to see the colors of my chakras. I focused my attention on the spots in my body where each chakra was supposed to be located starting at the top of my head. When I got to my second chakra I was immediately shown a circle made of bright orange carrots.

*I actually laughed out loud.* I wondered if I was hungry and my body was telling me something.

Then I realized that after I had seen the preceding chakra the color was yellow and I thought to myself *that the color was the same color of yellow as a banana.*

So, I got a response when I looked at the next chakra which was not only orange but matched my thought with a food, too. I mention this experience because, as I have learned, thoughts will also affect the aura.

So, be careful what you think about, because you are setting up thought forms in your aura.

Just think about this for a moment. And, remember what has happened around you that may have caused you to have a really good day verses a bad one. It could have been what you allowed yourself to give thought to.

*"There is only one good, knowledge, and one evil, ignorance."*
>—Socrates (469 BC–399 BC)
>*From Diogenes Laertius,*
>*Lives of Eminent Philosophers*

# 2

## *Aura Experiences*

I can't help but wonder, when I think back, if the following experience that I had in the early 1970's led me subconsciously on what appeared to be my search in answer to an unanswered medical question. That ended up helping me to discover more than I could ever have imaged about myself and the world within me as well as around me on ethereal levels.

One evening on my way to the gym as I was driving down the street I came to a traffic light that was red. I stopped my car, the light turned green and I drove through and then the street lights came on, as it was just becoming twilight. Then I realized that the street lights were green too. Then the headlights from all of the cars coming from the other direction were green, as well. I was really startled, since every light I was seeing was green. As soon as I could, I turned my car around and headed back home. I very carefully followed other vehicles until I reached my neighborhood and own driveway.

The next day I made an appointment with an eye doctor to have my vision checked. At the time I thought sure I must have some kind of impaired vision due to a medical problem. The ophthalmologist took every kind of test possible and found nothing wrong. My concern was that this could happen again and the next time I might not be so lucky when driving.

Almost twenty years later another instance would happen while I was having a conversation with a vice president when going over a funding proposal that I had drafted. When I looked down to pick up the proposal I saw what looked like a velvety liquid cobalt blue flowing down over the front of my body. Only this time I knew it was part of my aura because of all that I had read and experienced myself throughout the years.

I would come to learn a few years later, while living and working in the Pacific North West, when talking to a colleague who worked with the same organization of a very frightening experience she had when she saw her first aura, because she didn't know what it was.

She was attending a conference and had been taking notes during most of the lecture on that day, when she looked up quickly to view something that the speaker was showing on a chart and she saw a mixture of colors around the speaker. First, she saw a purple color running down the speaker's one arm—"it looked like paint being poured over him," she said. Then she saw yellow coming out of the middle of the speaker's body and there was an orange color right below it.

She was very fortunate when she went to see her family doctor that he had knowledge of the human aura and was therefore able to put her mind at ease. Her experience had encouraged her to learn about the human aura by reading whatever she could that had been written on the subject.

We both talked about her experience one day during lunch and I came to the conclusion that she was able to see the speaker's aura because of a poster she had been looking at in her office. It was the kind of poster that if you looked in between a blank space whatever was on the right and left side would form a complete picture. An example would be a divided tree becoming a whole tree. What she was doing was using both sides of her brain at once which I felt gave her extra energy in the center of her brain. This could have actually stimulated her third eye, the sixth chakra, her brow chakra.

*"You cannot acquire experience by making experiments. You cannot create experience. You must undergo it."*

—Albert Camus (1913–1960)
French existentialist author & philosopher

# 3

## *Seeing and Feeling Auras*

The brow chakra, also known as the spiritual eye, all seeing-eye, is what allows us to see the ethereal energies or subtle bodies. Everyone has seen some part of an aura during their life. Only they may not have known what it was.

If you have ever seen any little specks of color after being in the bright sunshine, they are usually blue, yellow, or pink you are probably seeing aspects of your aura or an aura that is near you. If you have ever seen a blue color around a house plant or an outside plant, you have seen an aura. Whenever you have seen a picture that has been taken of the earth from space there is usually a blue haze around it–that is the earth's aura. In fact, it appears that not only the earth but everything that is *of the earth* carries its signature which is blue, right next to the physical and where the ethereal energy begins.

Sometimes, depending on the time of day, especially at twilight, it is easy to see the outline of the aura from trees. At a distance and due to the light outside, the aura will look white and extend several feet out around the tops of the trees. The blue part of the aura is still there, but it is closer to the tree and is not easy to see from a distance.

One thing that might be of interest to the reader is to know that not all people see colors in the same way through the ethereal. Mainly because each of us are looking through our own auras which can often cast a different shade onto what we are viewing.

Remember earlier when I wrote about the colleague who saw a purple color running down the arm of the speaker who was giving the lecture? What she saw could have been the dark blue ethereal part of the speaker's aura that took on the color it did due to the colors in her own aura.

If you want to see auras here is a technique that might assist you in acquiring that ability. Put a live green plant on the right or left side—depending on which hand you use to apply your lipstick or shave your face—of a counter with a large mirror where you can see to apply your lipstick or when shaving. Think to yourself that you want to see an aura. As you are looking forward into the mirror, also use your peripheral vision (side vision) to look at the plant.

If you are right handed the plant will be on your right side and you will be looking with your side vision at the plant, or visa versa. You will eventually start to see a blue aura from the plant in the mirror as well as next to you. You will only be able to see it with your side vision. If you see it briefly and turn to look at it with your front vision it will be gone.

After you have seen the plants aura, you should be able to move to the next step in seeing an aura–your own. One way to get started is to look about two inches above your head for a couple of minutes, then look directly in the middle of your forehead, while gazing with a slightly out-of-focus relaxed vision in a mirror in dim light. You should start to see colors around your body after practicing this technique for five to ten minutes a day, over a two week period. Use the same mirror where you were able to see your plant's aura. Viewing your self while in the nude and having light colored walls around you will make it easier for you to see your aura, too. The larger the mirror, the more of your aura you will be able to see.

Again, since you are training your body it will already be conditioned to the process. You should also be thinking of what your intent is and that is to see your aura. At first, the colors will be very light and misty looking, but as you become more accustomed to seeing your aura you should be able to see more of its color.

When you have become experienced in seeing auras, you will be able to face any life-form and see an aura.

If you have a pet, you can also practice seeing its aura.

One way to get started is to first get used to what the aura feels like. By moving your hands down both sides of your pet's body at the same time in a sweeping motion, keeping them three to four inches away from its body, you should start to feel the form of its aura.

Once your pet realizes what you are doing, it will stand very still while you are doing this. In fact, you can use your hands to actually clear the aura of your pet when using this technique. One of my Dobermans, a female, used to love having her aura cleared.

Since one of your goals is to see auras remember to use your peripheral vision while using your hand-gliding technique. Also, out-of-focus vision will help you to see an aura more clearly. Since any aura is constantly changing in color and because it is constantly moving around you, you will only see it for brief moments at a time.

An interesting thing will start to happen once you are in tune with your pet's aura. You will start to feel your own aura more and will become more aware of the auras of those who are near you, which can be a good thing.

It is interesting how the ethereal level of energy works; it seems to open the door to other levels within your consciousness. You may even start to become aware of your own angels and guides, if they don't manifest physically before you in some way, they will often communicate with you through your third eye as Nicodemus did with me one evening as I made mention of in my book *Synchronicity*.

Getting back to pets and their auras, I have only been an owner of dogs and horses. But, I have fed stray cats. I learned a number of interesting things from these mystical creatures.

One thing is how, if they like you, they will roll around on their backs. This does not mean that they want you to pet them or even touch them. But, I was convinced when the stray cats that I had been feeding did this, they were releasing energies from the front of their bodies which in turn, was connecting to the energies of any person that was around them. They were connecting ethereally.

How clever I thought, since making this kind of connection would be a much stronger way for the cats to make an attachment than in any other way. By doing this their energy field was actually being in-parted on another energy field–whoever was next to them. Therefore, claiming it as their own in order to be fed the food that they wanted and needed in order to survive.

People make attachments too, through their aura, when they are close to another person's energy field. If you have ever been close to a person for very long and felt depleted of your energy they have probably taken some of your energy. Move away from anyone who has a habit of doing this.

Some people are good at dumping their troubles, too. Giving them to someone else by complaining and talking to such a degree that the other person actually takes on that same energy, what you have to do is to learn how to get the conversation moving in a more positive direction by changing the subject and doing more of the talking yourself. Then just break away from the whole situation as soon as you can.

Since everything is energy, then it is easy to see how energies can flow into or with other energies. Energy is also very easy to feel once you are aware of how it feels. Remember how the vortexes are twisting from a small pin-point in the physical body then actually form an open funnel out approximately two feet from the physical body? Anything near these funnels is mixing with other energies.

A good practice for protection is to stand at a slight angle instead of face-to-face with another person. Most people tend to do this without any conscious thought. But, be aware of the person who is bent on trying to face you no matter what, for s/he will, without realizing it, probably be trying to make a physical attachment to your energy field.

Used items such as books (from a library), antiques, used clothing, cars, and houses, anything that anyone else has touched will carry that person's energy. Energies can be eliminated by doing what Native American's have done throughout the centuries by smudging with dried herbs, which most health food stores will carry in their herb section. Smudging is also something you should do when buying any jewelry *new* or used.

One of my guides actually imparted his energy on a television set of mine, by touching it, because it was a way for him to connect more with me at that time. But, he was also able to create the problem with my television set so that I went for help.

Much like the elderly man, who was a helper in the grocery store, who held the only small bag of cat food left on the shelf, of that brand, before I brought it for the stray cats. He, too, had made a connection because his energy was left on the bag of cat food. In my book *Synchronicity*, I wrote about these experiences and other experiences in which my guides and angels made connections with me.

*"Facts are the enemy of the truth."*

—Don Quixote—*Man of La Mancha*

# 4

## *A Healthy Aura Means a Healthy Body*

I have learned over the years that when I see a dark speck or spot in my aura it means there is something in my energy field that doesn't belong. It appears as if a fly is buzzing around me. Whether it is a virus, bacteria, or even a negative thought-form, I get rid of it by visually encasing it in a bright white light until it is gone, or by smudging it out with white sage.

It's not too late to use these techniques even if whatever it is reaches the physical body by passing through the aura. The trick is to take action right away.

I can always tell if something should reach my physical body because it will show up like a shadow on the part of my body that is at risk. For example, I'll see a dark shadow around my nose on the side where a cold virus could be trying to attack. Then I take extra care to make sure I am getting the proper rest, as well as a proper amount of vitamin C, and I eat more raw fruits and vegetables to strengthen my body.

Wearing bright colors the same color as your chakras can also strengthen your body, as well as eating the same color of foods as your chakras.

Any daily physical exercise, in which you are moving your entire body continuously, for at least a half an hour, will help to keep the energy flowing throughout your body, chakras and aura. All three must be in balance so that health and harmony can be achieved.

Jewelry, stones, crystals, and that extra change that you may be carrying around in a pocket, as well as any kind of metal that is on clothing, all affect the body's energy field. When going to bed at night your body should be free from all of these since they could cause imbalances and even holes in an aura. When holes and breaks happen to an aura the physical body has no protection, it's like having an open wound on your body without a bandage.

Holes in an aura can also take place if a serious injury happens to the physical body. What this means is that there would be a break in the energy field surrounding the physical body. If you cannot feel or see your own aura to smooth it out, it is possible to have the aura repaired by a therapist who can feel or see auras. Some massage therapists can feel auras even if they are not able to see them, and would be able to help repair any damages.

In this case the therapist would not work with the physical body, but would actually be touching the energy field that surrounds the body by gliding his/her hands over it, much like painting brush strokes. This kind of technique helps to reconnect any separations/holes that have been made. It may take more than one treatment, but immediate results will be felt in the physical body and the healing process of the physical body will be sped up.

*"All the world's a stage, and all the men and women merely players. They have their exits and their entrances, and one man in his time plays many parts."*

—William Shakespeare (1564–1616),
*As You Like It*
Greatest English dramatist & Poet

# 5

## *Energy Patterns*

The guides and angels that I mentioned in my book *Synchronicity*, who came through to help me, also affected the energy pattern of other things around those locations, too:

When Archangel Michael first came through to me there was a very heavy rain storm that took place as I was leaving the lecture. Local farmers were in need of rain at that time for their spring crops, so they benefited.

After Nicodemus came through on his bike, within a short time the officials in the village where we met, and the next town, decided to build a bikeway adjoining the two locations.

And, a walk-over wooden bridge was built, within a year, over the stream that I stood in and walked across, where I was greeted by another one of my guides.

After I met Forrest, another guide, at the Glen, he actually changed some planetary energy pattern within the Glen. And, at the same time, was communicating with me on another level about the energy patterns within me which he was changing, too.

A local health food store was asked to move by the property owners to a better location after being in the same location for over thirty years. This move took place several years after a couple of my guides had made contact with me within the store.

After interacting with another one of my guides at the local recycle center, within a two year period the entire drop-off center was moved, from its over twenty-five year location, to another location that was a modern up-scale center.

I find it very interesting how the *energy patterns* from my guides and angels have affected so many different *levels* of energy in such positive ways. And, I also can't help but wonder how others who may have been near them when they were actually helping me could have benefited in some way, too.

My angels and guides are truly miracle workers. And, I love seeing the magic that takes place when they are doing their work.

If I only knew how often they have actually saved my life I know I would really realize just how blessed I am. However, I am keenly aware of one time when I had a vision during the night.

What I saw was so startling to me that I woke up very frightened. I saw a huge set of horns (antlers) right in front of me, and a winding bright red ribbon-like form twisting around below it. Immediately I asked for more help. I was not given any more information in a vision and I didn't know what was going to happen. But, whatever it was scared me so much I had trouble going back to sleep.

It was winter-time in the Midwest and it was still dark when I drove to work at 7AM the next morning. As I was driving past an arboretum, which has over six hundred acres of trails and wooded areas with a large number of wild-life habitats, I heard the sound of hoofs near my car. I immediately took my foot off of the gas pedal. Then I saw something very large move by the window of the passenger's side of the car. It was a buck (male deer) that I am sure would have measured at least 15 hands high from its withers (highest part of his back). His height including his neck and head with antlers would have put him somewhere around seven or eight feet in total height. He proceeded to cross right in front of my car and ran across five lanes to the other side of the road. I missed him by inches. He was blessed many times over as other vehicles coming from both directions gave him a path as he sailed through the air and on into a wooded area.

Then I remembered the vision that I had been given during the night. What had looked like a bright red ribbon was really a *potentially* bloody road way. I know if I had not been given this vision during the night, which was still in my subconscious, there was a good chance that I would have hit the deer since I never had time to apply the brakes. So, my guides not only saved the life of a deer, but possibly mine too, as well as others who were driving in the area on that morning.

As I continued my drive into the city, this incident reminded me of the time when I was in my early twenties. I had just parked my car in a parking lot and was walking across the lot when a driver of a car immediately in front of me threw his car in reverse and backed-up at a very high speed. I felt the breeze from the car pass behind me as I actually jumped forward on the one foot I had on the ground at the time, since I didn't have time to even take another step to get out-of-the-way. I remember at the time how light by body felt. It was as if I was being lifted-up by another force.

◆    ◆    ◆

Another bit of magic was created recently which involved the actual *manifestation* of an additional architectural blue print which was found by one of the mover's who was placing office furniture and files in a newly renovated area where I worked.

The original blue print showed all of the filing cabinets placed in an open hallway and not in any of the offices. I pointed this out to the director, at the time, who said that he had no recourse but to follow what was shown on the blue print.

I also pointed this error out to another colleague, who said he would mention the situation to the director, too. The end result of both conversations was that "no changes were to be made." And, any changes that would need to be made would take place at a later date, after everything was in place as indicated on the blue print. So, all of the filing cabinets for everyone were virtually placed in an open hallway.

The next day one of the movers called me and said he didn't know what to do since his blue print did not match an area that was already set-up. As I walked into the area where he was, I instantly felt a difference in the energy around him from the day before. He was very jovial as I walked up to him, saying to me as we walked down the hallway together "come into my office I want to show you something."

When we reached the end of the hall he pulled a copy of a blue print from on top of one of the file cabinets and said, "this blue print shows these files should be in other places," as he pointed to the draft.

I took a double-take, since I had seen the original blue print, and he was right, this blue print, the one I was looking at actually showed all of the filing cabinets were where they were supposed to be in each of the offices. I called the director, who after seeing this latest blue print authorized the move saying that he must have misread the blue print the day before. The story doesn't end here.

A few days later when the manager responsible for the move was talking to the director, I overheard the director saying that he wanted to show him why there were changes made in the moving of the filing cabinets.

When the director took the blue print that was left on the shelf in the hallway it showed the cabinets the way they were when he first saw it, all of the filing cabinets were shown together in the hallway. Again, he thought he had misread the blue print. But, the move was already made. The second blue print was never found, and everyone assumed that the mover must have taken it with him.

I know from the energy field that I felt around the mover, who wanted me to see his blue print, that one of my guides had actually worked through the mover and created another blue print that showed the filing cabinets where they really belonged for my office and for everyone else's office, too.

♦ ♦ ♦

It was late September, 2006, and my first book was already at the publishers or this experience would have been a part of that book, too.

I was at the gym using a pull-down bar of weights when a tall dark haired male, who looked to be in his late 30's, sat down in the row of exercise equipment in front of me to use the same type of equipment that I was using. I noticed him looking at me through the mirror in front of him that lined the wall.

It was then that he made an adjustment to his watch then pulled down the bar that held the weights. I watched as the muscle rippled on the upper part of his arm leaving a bulge with each pull. For some reason, I felt that he wanted me to see him doing his exercises.

*But, why, I wondered? And, who was this guy?*

Then I left the pull-down bar and went over to the kick-back machine that tones the back of the leg and lower-back.

It was then that he walked in front of me, smiled and said, "Hello."

*Hello*, I said, and smiled back at him. His energies felt liquid to me as he walked by.

I watched him as he continued to walk by and around the end of the rest of the equipment in the row where I was exercising and then he actually walked behind me and on down to the other end of the room.

It was then that I realized he looked just like a colleague who I had congratulated on having becoming a doctor several years prior. It was also then that I realized this was a guide with some kind of message and I needed to really pay attention. But, when I looked again in the direction where he was walking, he was gone.

Now each time I went to the gym I looked for him. But, knowing how angels and my guides' work I thought the chances of my seeing this same image that he projected again would be slim.

Then on October 3, 2006 while at the gym, it happened. I was laughing out loud at the way one of the trainers was trying to help one of the clubs members, when a young man who looked to be in his twenties, a very small person with light hair, who didn't look familiar to me at all, and who was using some equipment next to me, started laughing, too.

And, he said, "That trainer is so funny isn't he."

I said, *yes he is.*

Then he asked, "would you show me how to use that equipment you are using? There is nothing like it where I come from."

I said, *sure. Are you visiting from the gym south of here?* My question seemed to make him nervous and he squirmed around in his seat.

He replied, "I'm not from around here."

I said, *oh.* Then I proceeded to show him how to adjust the bar in front of me, the foot rest, and the weights and followed through by bending from my waist in a forward motion. This equipment was to exercise the front and back of the torso. Then I realized he was gone.

So, again I was left trying to figure out what was the real message? And, what did I need to know? What did I need to do?

I thought and thought and I had concluded that it had something to do with health because the first guide that I saw made himself look like a doctor that I knew. Also, this same doctor had a great sense of humor and always made me laugh, so again the second guide brought this information through. *Boy, do I ever hate playing charades!*

But, I still couldn't figure out what the real message was. Then I saw it, one evening when I had opened up the refrigerator door and I was reaching in with my left arm to get something I noticed a lump on the inside of my arm.

*That's it, I said out loud!*

It was a tumor and it appeared to be like what I had removed several years earlier from my lower back. Completely harmless, slow growing, and in most cases the kind that some people never have removed, according to what I had heard from one medical person.

I quickly went to my doctor and she told me "yes" it was a fatty tumor like what I had had removed from my back, and, not to worry, they were slow growing and harmless. Still I didn't want it in my body.

That night while in bed with my eyes closed I asked what the solution in getting rid of it was. I saw three images in a vertical line. The first, at the top was a very small tumor, (much smaller than what was on my arm); the second was a tumor about three times as big. Then I saw a cluster of people wearing white robes and white masks in an operating room in a circle (as if I was up in the air looking down on them).

I immediately said *no,* I don't want another operation by human beings, have my guides or angels take it away. I am still waiting! But, the tumor is getting smaller. And, every time I look at it I say "dissolve it," then I close my eyes and see it as a tiny speck.

Tumors are caused by toxins in the body and I know that I cannot take very many vitamins or supplements because they can affect my body adversely. I also know the dangers of hydrogenated oils which I never use myself, but I cannot be sure that I am not getting them when I eat out in a restaurant, even if they claim they don't use them.

I am so grateful to my guides for coming into my *energy field* and making me aware of what needs to be done to help keep my body healthy.

*"The unexamined life is not worth living."*
—Socrates (469 BC–399 BC),
*In Plato, Dialogues,*
*Apology*

# 6

## *Cause and Affect: Thoughts Create Actions*

Thoughts usually come before any actions. By this I mean usually a thought is given to or about something before any action is taken. A person will have thoughts about going somewhere on a trip before making the trip. A person will think about having some chocolate before actually eating any.

When this happens, you are actually cultivating whatever it is you are thinking about through your thoughts. I mentioned earlier the importance of what thought is, and how it affects the body's aura, because thoughts can actually take form over time. Yes, thought-forms do exist in the ethereal energy field.

By changing your thoughts you can change your aura, body, and your entire life. This has been proven over-and-over again by people who have been healed physically, mentally, and emotionally just by the way they think.

The first step in changing thoughts is to become aware of what you are thinking about, this is not an easy thing to do, when you stop and think about it, because we are constantly thinking. Even when we are sleeping, there are so many electrical impulses playing out in our brains from the days activities that by the time most people get up in the morning from a night's rest they have barely unwound from the preceding day's activities.

I know that I always feel much better when I have remembered a dream or two during my night's sleep. This tells me a couple of things. One, I am connecting to who I am, and two, that I am rested enough to be able to remember what I have dreamt about.

The thoughts of others can affect the way you feel, too. I am sure this is of no great surprise to anyone, since everyone during sometime in their life knows what it feels like to have a very angry, sad, or ill person near them.

But, since energy can travel great distances, it is also possible to be affected by someone's thoughts about you, good or bad. Again what comes into play here is the ethereal realm.

Keep this in mind if you are feeling a little out-of-sorts. And, if you think about what you are feeling long enough you should be able to figure out who the energy is coming from. Then you can confront the person by visualizing their face in your mind and telling them to stop their negative thoughts. This always works because you are reaching them through their subconscious.

However, in time, even if you do not use this approach, usually one of your angels will have made contact with one of the person's angels, and the whole situation will be cast aside. You will know this too, by the way that you start to feel again.

◆ ◆ ◆

It was through my own thoughts that I asked my angels/guides about a beloved deceased Doberman of mine. I remember thinking one evening right before going to sleep how much I missed him and that I hoped he was doing okay wherever he was, and that I would really like to see him.

It was a day or two later, just as daylight was breaking, that I heard him running through the dinning room, into the hallway, sliding around corners, the sound of his feet hitting the hardwood floor, and then entering my bedroom barking. There was a slight brush of his body against the side of my bed, the sound of children laughing, and then he paused briefly next to my bed, gave a few whimpers and then the angel children called him by his name and said "come on, let's go." They all actually exited through the closed window in my bedroom. This time I did not see him or the angel children; I only heard them.

He has come to visit me two more times—almost a decade apart. One time was after I had been around other dogs, and another time after I had seen someone walking a Doberman down the street. Each time I had been thinking of him prior to his visits. During both of these times, I was sleeping as I heard his whimper and then felt him lick my face. I saw him only briefly as I opened my eyes one of those times. Then he was gone as quickly as he came.

I know this dear pet is really around more times than I am aware, because I have sensed him during times when I happen to be out walking at night, or in situations where I might feel uncomfortable in a certain setting. My awareness of him is as if he is sending me thoughts letting me know that he is with me.

His thoughts will then remind me of the time he scared off an intruder who came knocking at my front door one night at 11:00pm. When I opened the shutters to the window next to the front door, the young male intruder saw a giant of a Doberman. His eyes became as big as saucers and he left quickly.

I would imagine that my deceased Doberman would probably send some kind of a frightening thought to anyone who would try to cause any harm to me; there-by, changing their intentions for any wrong doing. Much like the way my angels and guides would work.

Animals are very telepathic anyway. My experience with the cats in my book *Synchronicity* is a good example of this. It was really interesting how their thoughts kept getting through to me with pictures during the night while I was sleeping. I would see an actual image of whichever one would be around the next day or even which one would be outside during the night waiting to see me or to get some more food. It took me a while to realize that one of the cats, the white-and-gray spotted one, was sending me mental messages for his personal feeding schedule, which was every morning at 6:30am. Yes, I was actually getting up at 6:30am every day to feed him. And, I was also feeding him every evening.

When I would try to sleep past 6:30am on the weekends, I would continually have visions while sleeping where I would see him outside curled-up waiting for me to bring him his food. When I would arrive with his food, I would get an expression of loving gratitude which would involve a few very slow blinks with his eyes.

He never would come close to his food until I was several feet away from him. This white-and-gray spotted cat I felt belonged to the elderly man I saw in the grocery store; who was, I believe, a good wizard, who would appear in a second and disappear the next, or not show his physical self, but I often felt his presence when he was near the cat.

So, I began to wonder if it really was the cats or was it the good wizard who was sending me the mental visions. Was this a kind of training to help me be more aware of him?

Was he the good wizard who had been helping me since the mid 1980's when I found the pieces of broken clay flower pots next to the water faucets outside my house as a sign to add more live plants inside my house?

I know that each of my guides and angels have had their own way of interacting with me, and when I think about their interactions with me, it has been like playing a game of charades.

It doesn't seem to matter how I react with them, because they always do what they have intended to do no-matter-what, which is to help me even if I'm not aware of what the help is at the time. It's something I am usually able to conclude after-the-fact, which is probably the way they want it, since they often will make themselves look different so I won't recognize them.

Or, could it have something to do with them impinging on my free will or my attitude? And what has been established in a universal law in the spiritual realm that they must follow, to comply with—help without interfering with a person's free will.

So, their interaction with me gives me the awareness to do something that I otherwise may not have known or thought about doing, but in the end will take my own action to do it, because an angel or guide has planted the seed.

Like the time I decided to quit smoking cigarettes on an Easter Sunday. It seems like everything I have ever done in my life that took a great deal of *will power* always took place on an Easter Sunday.

However, as strange as this may sound I would not realize that the process had really started on Easter until after-the-fact.

Smoking tobacco is an addiction. It not only burns up all of the vitamin A in your body, it leaves the same kind of sticky residue in your aura as it does within your body and on everything around you.

I myself have not been able to see this residue within any aura, but one time when I heard a Shaman give a talk she mentioned that this sticky residue could be pulled out of the aura and once it was removed a person would not have the desire to smoke again.

In fact, she had smoked for a number of years and it was another Shaman who removed the residue from her aura and stopped her from smoking. Since then, anytime she was around anyone who smoked she would become very sick, and would have to leave the area.

I wish I had known her at the time I was trying to quit because it was a real nightmare for me to get through it at that time. There were times when I would run into doors and doorways and stumble around as if I was in a daze. Then I would realize that I was holding my breath–I needed oxygen.

Why? Because I had been a chain smoker and smoked three packs of cigarettes a day. A good portion of every breath that I had been used to taking was to inhale smoke. My breathing in-and-out was controlled by the number of cigarettes I was smoking.

When I first began to smoke it didn't come naturally. In fact, I didn't even like it, but within a short period of time I was enjoying every single puff, and I wanted more, and more. I only started smoking because it was the "in" thing to do at the time.

I remember during those years when I did smoke how I always had trouble seeing clearly at night when I was driving. After I quit smoking, my night vision was perfect again.

The only way I was able to stop smoking was to change everything that I could that I did when I smoked, which was everything, since I was a chain smoker. Following are some examples that might be helpful to you or someone that you know.

I stopped drinking coffee in the morning and evening since these were times when I would naturally smoke, too.

I stopped reading the paper in the morning, and read it later in the day, since this was also a time when I would usually smoke.

As soon as I was finished with a meal I would use my cigarette-holder as a prop. I would pretend that I was having a cigarette. Then I would get up from the table as soon as I could. Wait twenty minutes and take a walk for a half an hour.

I joined a local gym to keep my thoughts on something else. I worked out seven days a week in addition to walking a half an hour three times every day.

Once the cravings were so strong I bought a pack of cigarettes telling myself to just smell the tobacco and pretend to smoke, but don't light up. I was successful! I ended up chewing on the tips of the cigarettes until I reached the tobacco and then would throw it away. I went through several cartons this way.

My next step was to use cut-up celery sticks, cut to the same size as a cigarette. I would carry these with me wherever I went. I realized that from having smoked for a decade I had cultivated an oral hand-to-mouth habit in addition to taking a drag (deep breath) from a cigarette that somehow had become a stress releaser. So, I applied the same thought process to the celery sticks.

It was working. Only it turned out to be a bit tricky when I was in meetings. One day a fellow colleague wanted to know what the green thing was that I seemed to be trying to inhale. So, I confessed that it was my cigarette made from celery. He wanted to know where he could get one. Then we both laughed.

The hardest part about trying to stop smoking was whenever I would go to parties. So, I always made sure to take my cigarette-holder so I would have something to hold on to and not drink any alcoholic beverages or coffee. This was very calming since the smell of cigarettes was in the holder.

I really struggled for over a year, and then it happened. I remember very clearly waking up one morning with the taste of cigarettes in my mouth, and I remembered being at a party, I thought, the night before. But, wait a minute, as I sat up on the edge of my bed, the alarm went off and I realized I had only had a dream about having smoked, but it seemed so real for a brief moment.

This would be the first of many more dreams that I would have thinking that I had smoked at a party. Each time I would be so disappointed with myself until I would realize the truth.

By the end of my second year without a cigarette, the cravings were gone and replaced with a zest to do all of the right things for myself physically, mentally, spiritually, and emotionally. This is something that has become a way of life for me today.

Change just *one thought* in your life or change just *one thing* in your life and you can transform who you are on many different levels.

You may also become aware of levels of consciousness within you that you never knew existed.

*What if you slept?*

*And what if in your sleep you dreamed? And what if in your dream you went to heaven, and there plucked a strange and beautiful flower? And what if when you awoke you had the flower in your hand?*

*Ah, what then?*

—Samuel Taylor Coleridge
*English critic & poet (1772–1834)*

# 7

## *Dreams, Past Lives, or Night Travels?*

We've all had them—dreams! But how do we know if they are really dreams or an event from a past life? Or, for that matter, something that our mind has created in a picture as a response to what we are feeling or thinking at a certain time, or even something else.

Well, usually when I dream, I am able to connect it to something that I am aware of in my life; an event, situation, person or place.

Whenever I have had an experience that I felt was connected to a past life I am usually shown an image of myself, by myself, standing in the middle of a spotlight, as if I am on a stage, looking at myself, face-to-face. And, the message that I am left with depends on what my spirit is trying to show me about my soul; soul meaning that which I am made up from all of my past lives.

One example of this was when I saw myself as a female with light colored hair and very light skin. I appeared to be tall and slender, since I seemed to be looking up at my stature as it was then. A facial expression of a shy timid person was shown to me, yet smiling in a submissive way.

As I was looking at this image I got a very strong feeling that I was being shown a life that was oppressive and abusive, almost as if being confined like a prisoner–helpless, a person who did not know how to help herself on any level in any way. The image made me feel weak and sick at my stomach.

Yet, the image was gone as soon as it came. My mind immediately flashed to the person that I had been dating. A person who I had sensed right up front was very controlling, for one thing, there were other things, too, that didn't feel right about him.

Although he was probably one of the most handsome, interesting, wealthy and well educated young men I had ever dated. I stopped dating him, however, something was off! And, I didn't want to stick around to find out what it was.

I have been shown many other images of my past lives, and while I never looked exactly the same, I was always able to sense that it was me that I was being shown and then an impression was left for the reason(s) why.

Like the time I had been reading an article one evening about a certain political person in power at the time in England, and how during that night while in bed I was again face-to-face with myself looking at a female who wore a turban-like hat that was weaved out of a fabric that was mostly green with flecks of other colors in it, whose deep-set dark colored eyes and her face held an expression of such depth and great power that I was startled. There was no question in my mind that it was me and I held some kind of powerful position during that life-time. I was left with the feeling that many were fearful of me then, and I was not one for anyone to try and fool with on any level.

Then there are the pictures that my mind creates, which are always in color, that can be precipitated by me, an angel, or one of my guides, as a message while I am awake or asleep. They come as images through my brow chakra (third eye) in the middle of my forehead. If I am using my two physical eyes I will see an image through my third eye. The image from this single eye will either give me a quick flash of an image or a series of images.

I have to be paying attention because there are no instant replays, only different kinds of images or nothing at all. One example of this was when I saw in a flash, to my right, in the middle of the street, several men in work-clothes as I was taking a walk one afternoon. Only there were no men actually there at that time. Instead, they were there the next day doing some street repairs when I was taking a walk. When I saw them from a distance I turned and went in the opposite direction, since I thought there must have been a reason why I had gotten an earlier vision of them.

The other kind of images that my mind creates, or are given to me by angels or my guides, can look like pieces of clip art. Like the image of the young girl I saw who said her name was Elizabeth that I mentioned in my book *Synchronicity*. And fragments of pictures or places as a message like the vision, I mentioned earlier in this book, that I was given during the night about seeing antlers and what looked like red ribbon, which turned out the next day to be the deer I encountered in the roadway on my way to work.

◆ ◆ ◆

There are other kinds of visions that I have only had during the night. These are visions where I actually find myself looking down at the earth from high in the sky, or I am watching an event, or I am watching myself doing something in which I am not able to identify as a dream, past life, or some kind of night travel when I am asleep.

One time, during the night, I was aware of a male's voice saying to me just as I was about to go to sleep, "come on, let's go." That's all I remember. But the feeling that I had at that moment was we had to be somewhere fast and we could not afford to be late.

The following experiences have only happened when I have been vacationing on several islands, and while I have been to other islands, I don't remember having experiences like what I have had while visiting the U.S. Virgin Islands, Bermuda, and Martha's Vineyard. Each time I would be waking up in the morning from a night's sleep and would be up so high in the sky that I could see the entire island, and then I would be aware that I was still in bed and awake. The feelings that went along with this were calmness and a great sense of peace, until I was fully awake.

I was really made aware of the energies in the earth of each of these islands, too. And, I was very glad to leave Bermuda. Even though it was visually the most beautiful of the three islands, the energies were really off. I felt fragmented while there, and I realized this even more the second time I visited. At that time I thought, *I never want to come back here again.* The energies seemed to be the polar opposite of those I have since experienced in Sedona, AZ.

A frequent event that I have seen while sleeping is when I am walking in a very lush jungle and there are wild animals around me, but the only thing I see is a wild bore running on a path in front of me. I can sense that there are other animals near, but I am not afraid because I know that they cannot harm me. And, they also know that I won't harm them. It's as if I have come to look at the environment in the jungle, which always looks lush and healthy and everything seems to be in balance. I can smell the fresh damp earth and a scent from some fragrant plant; it's sweet, yet pungent. Its fragrance always reminds me of something at the time when I am there, but I can never seem to remember what once I leave the jungle and I am awake.

This dream, past life, or some kind of travel-at-night while my body is sleeping experience, I have seen off-and-on since I was a very young child. I am walking down a moss lined path in a forest, in my bare feet, wearing a long night gown. I can see the sunlight shining down through the dense tree lined path. The weather is warm, like summertime.

I can feel the soft powdered dirt on the bottoms of my feet; it's warm and dry and puffs up into the air with each step that I take. I love the way it feels, I reach down and take a handful of it. Then, I carry it with me as I walk, but soon it disappears from my hand.

Now I am walking on moss which seems to cover most of the path; it's soft too. Its cool compared to the powdered dirt. I have a struggling thought within my mind as to which I like the best the powdery dirt or the moss. I can't decide. Then I wonder why I have to make a choice. *Why should one be better than the other?*

I am now aware of the giant trees that have blocked out most of the sunlight from the path. For a brief moment I feel afraid. Then I hear birds chirping and see them flying along next to me in the trees. The path is long but I never get tired. Then I see it. The small cottage that I go to and visit with a lady who answers all of my questions.

She is very tall, or seems tall since I am so small, with very long blonde hair. She is always loving, kind, and gentle. When we are together she reminds me of all of the things that I am supposed to do when I grow-up. None of them have to do with raising a family. They are other things that she shows me in pictures with her mind, when I am looking at her face, but I have trouble knowing what they mean.

She always tells me to trust how I feel and all of the pictures will have the right meanings for me in the end. And, to always remember that she and her friends would be showing me more pictures even when I don't come to visit her after I have grown-up.

As I continued to grow-up I had trouble finding my way through the forest. I kept taking wrong paths; I could not find the small cottage that I often visited. Then I forgot about it, and something within felt missing and I didn't know where to go to even look for what I felt I had lost.

I looked in all kinds of areas, and within all kinds of other people, but the void only grew. I wondered, *was I having growing pains?*

◆ ◆ ◆

Then when I was a teenager there was a kind of awareness that took place. During the night when I would be thinking about something, like a jacket in a certain color, that I wanted and I hoped I could find to buy I would then, during that night, actually see myself in the jacket.

I continued to see pictures of myself doing different things at school and with friends during the night when I was sleeping. And, this same process continued throughout my twenties. I thought I was having dreams. But, it would not be until my mid-twenties that I would realize that I was having visions of things before they would actually happen. My whole awareness was heightened in the techniques of visual awareness after taking yoga classes. Then I attained an even greater awareness after angels and my guides began to interact with me as described in my book *Synchronicity*.

Since guides and angels can use any object they choose, besides themselves, they were using everything they could to continually communicate with me on every level possible day and night.

I heard them, I saw them, I felt them, but I didn't know who they were until I had experienced complete synchronicity. This was the real break through.

It was the missing link that enabled a shift to take place within my consciousness and helped opened the door to my awareness. And, I am sure that I will continue to know and experience even more than I could have ever imagined.

We are far more than what our human eyes are able to see. But, once we are connected to our own spiritual side—and this can happen in a number of ways—then a very magical life can unfold before us.

*"The most beautiful experience we can have is the mysterious."*
—Albert Einstein (1879–1955)
*US (German-born) physicist*

# 8

## *Magic in the Air*

*Often, whenever an angel or one of my guides appears, there has been a kind of magic in the air.*

It's the kind of feeling that I get during the Christmas holidays when there seems to be a joyfulness everywhere, with an anticipation that something very special is about to happen.

This feeling of magic seems to depend on where my thoughts are at the time. If I am not thinking about anything or preoccupied with something at the time when angels and my guides are around me, then I am aware of them in my energy field.

I can be aware of this magical feeling before angels and my guides appear, and after they have gone. But, the amazing thing is that I am *not always* aware of them at the very moment they are interacting with me.

Angels and my guides only come to help, but they don't come by just to say hello, and they always have a message. It's as if they each have a certain responsibility, commitment. Some may be responsible for my safety, some for physical, mental, or spiritual support and others for healings on all levels.

Usually my guides and angels that I see in person are male. But, when I was very young I felt the energies around me were more from female guides and angels.

Since becoming an adult, the only female guide I can remember seeing is the one that I have seen during the night, when I have had visions of a very beautiful young women with long dark hair down to her waist, wearing a long white gown. She is usually walking in front of me, and I only see her back, but the one time when I saw her facing me she was in a very windy place, and she was showing me an image that included a virtual picture of all of my chakras, and each one was very bright and colorful. At the time, I never understood the message.

Each time I have seen an angel or one of my male guides they have imparted something to me from them, like courage, faith, forthrightness, joy, and a healthy stronger energy field and physical body.

Also, I am left with an over-all feeling that what is here in this life is such a very small part of who I really am, and the best part is yet to come.

978-0-595-43627-9
0-595-43627-7